Balance and Your Body

Also by Amanda Sterczyk

*Move More, Your Life Depends On It:
Practical Tips to Add More Movement to Your Day*
(CreateSpace Independent Publishing Platform, 2018).

Balance and Your Body

How Exercise Can Help You Avoid a Fall

Amanda Sterczyk

Foreword by Robert H. Wood

The information in this book should not be used for diagnosis or treatment, or as a substitute for professional medical care. Before beginning any exercise program, consult your physician.

Copyright © Amanda Sterczyk 2019
Foreword © Robert Wood 2019

All rights reserved. No part of this publication may be reproduced, stored in a retrieval system or transmitted in any form or by any means without the prior written permission of the author, nor be otherwise circulated in any form of binding or cover other than that in which it is published and without a similar condition being imposed on the purchaser.

Excerpt from *You CAN Prevent Falls!* Public Health Agency of Canada. Adapted and reproduced with permission from the Minister of Health, 2019. © All rights reserved.

Excerpt from "Why Seniors Fall," published by *Electronics Caregiver* © 2012 Robert Wood. Reproduced with permission. All rights reserved.

Excerpt from "How I felt after 70 days of lying in bed for science," *Vice Magazine* © 2015 Andrew Iwanicki. Reproduced with permission. All rights reserved.

Excerpt from *One Heart, Two Feet: Enhancing Heart Health, One Step at a Time*, published by Creative Walking, © 2016 Barry Franklin and Robert Sweetgall. Reproduced with permission. All rights reserved.

Excerpt from *Fact Sheet on Physical Activity*, published by World Health Organization © 2014. Used with permission. All rights reserved.

Sterczyk, Amanda, author
    Balance and Your Body: How Exercise Can Help You Avoid a Fall / Amanda Sterczyk.

Includes bibliographical references.
Issued in print and electronic formats.

ISBN 9781072499251

    1. Aging. 2. Fall Prevention 3. Physical Fitness 4. Healthy Aging 5. Balance Training

Editor: Kaarina Stiff
Cover: Dianna Little, cover image: iStock Photo
Exercise Illustrations: Emily Sterczyk
Layout: Matthew Bin
Proofreading: Rhys Jennings
Author photo: Allison Mundle
Published by Kindle Direct Publishing

May you live a long and healthy life,
free from slips, trips, and broken hips.
And falls.

Move more, feel better.

CONTENTS

Foreword	9
Introduction	11
Part One: The Problem	**15**
Fear of Falling	17
Is Fear a Vicious Circle?	17
Have You Ever Fallen?	18
What's the Problem with Falling?	19
Exercise vs. Getting in Shape	23
Are You in Shape?	23
How Much and What Type of Exercise Do You Need?	25
Are There Benefits to Light Physical Activity?	27
Balance and Gravity	29
How's Your Balance?	29
Do You Know about the Heel-Toe Express?	31
What's Gravity Got to Do With It?	32
Part Two: The Solution	**35**
Fall Prevention	37
Want to Hear About My First Encounter with Fall Prevention?	37
Have You Seen Fall Prevention Programs Lately?	38
Can You Regain Your Confidence after a Fall?	39
Balance Basics	41
Do You Know the Three Pillars of Balance?	41
Is It a Photo or a Video?	43
Can You Improve Your Balance in Three Days?	44
How's Your Walking?	46
Balance and Strength	49
Have You Ever Tripped Over Your Own Foot?	49
What Does It Mean to Exercise?	50
Will Those Stairs Really Kill You?	51
Can You Do a Side Shuffle?	53
Balance and Posture	55
How Does Your Posture Impact Your Fall Risk?	55
Do You Play the Piano?	56
Do You Window Shop?	58
Are You a Comma, Question Mark, or Exclamation Point?	59
Balance and Your Joints	61
Are Your Ankles Stiff?	61

Are You a Well-Oiled Machine?	62
Do You Play with CARs?	63
Part Three: The Action Plan	**65**
Functional Fitness	**67**
Does Practice Make Perfect?	67
What's Functional Fitness?	68
Do You Know How to Turn a Movement into Exercise?	69
Can We Talk About Safety?	70
The Exercises	**73**
Tackling the Exercises One at a Time	73
Before You Begin	74
Definitions	75
Finger Follow	78
Static Balance	80
Clock Toe Taps	82
Dynamic Walking	84
Lower Body Strength Exercises	86
High March	87
Heel Raises	88
Counter Squats	89
Four-Way Hip Strengthener	90
Sideways Walking	92
Active Sitting	94
Active Standing	96
Joint Mobility	98
Ankles	99
Knees	100
Hips	101
Waist	102
Fingers	103
Wrists	104
Elbows	105
Shoulders	106
Neck	107
Notes	**109**
Acknowledgements	**115**
Reviews of *Move More, Your Life Depends On It*	**117**
About the Author	**119**

FOREWORD

I first had the pleasure to meet Amanda when she was working on her first book, *Move More, Your Life Depends On It: Practical Tips to Add More Movement to Your Day*. As we chatted over Skype about some of the content of this first text, it became clear to me that Amanda is very passionate about serving the needs of the community. She is also very thoughtful and careful about ensuring the validity of the scientific evidence that she uses to support her work. It also struck me that Amanda is gifted at presenting the scientific underpinnings of complex topics, such as balance, in language that can be easily understood and resonates with readers. Because of her passion for her work, Amanda connects very easily with readers and skillfully brings important concepts to light.

Ultimately, this text, *Balance and Your Body*, is an effort to break the debilitating cycle of the "fear of falling." This is a complex milieu of psychological and physical alterations that can occur with age and age-related diseases. The fear of falling also involves fearing the implications of reporting a fall, with many seniors worrying, "Will my independence be taken from me?"

As we age and our balance and postural stability become compromised, we are less likely to engage in certain otherwise healthy activities that we believe could pose a threat to our ability to maintain our balance, not just because of potential physical injury, but because we wish to avoid these other implications. However, when we avoid situations that challenge our balance, we miss opportunities to optimize our physical function, which further exacerbates the problem.

In this book, Amanda taps into the "fear of falling" in a way that captures many of our experiences, and subsequently, the concerns that arise as we age. She connects with readers' conceptions, and sometimes misconceptions, and thereby draws attention to the opportunities we all have to age successfully and to optimize our functional lifespan. She provides guidance for readers based on solid scientific evidence to assist with safe and effective activities that reduce the risk of falls. By connecting with readers and offering safe and effective opportunities, Amanda's work will positively impact the lives of many adults who are struggling with balance issues. This work will add to the quality of life in the community, which is clearly her passion.

Robert H. Wood, PhD
Director, School of Allied Health
Boise State University

INTRODUCTION

We all have a "physical" best-before date. Hopefully, we are able to live fully and enjoy life before our bodies hit that date. As we age and our bodies begin to decline, many people experience difficulty with simple tasks. What we don't want — well, at least what I don't want, and I hope you want the same thing — is to live through years or decades of infirmity before we die. I want to live well until my time is up, which is why I keep physical activity on my daily to-do list.

What's on your bucket list? Do you worry that you're missing out on things because of your physical activity level? Has a fear of falling or a past fall impacted how and when you go out? As we get older, the risk of falls that can injure us increases. As a result, individuals just like you curb their activity levels. But it doesn't have to be that way. If you take charge of your body, you can be as active as you like.

Working on improving your balance and strengthening your muscles will increase your confidence and reduce the risk of a fall. So you can get back to enjoying your life, and continue to tackle that bucket list, enjoy life, and live fully each day.

How Does a Child View Seniors?

I grew up with seniors in my circle. In addition to spending time with my immediate family, I frequently visited my elderly maternal grandparents and two great-aunts. I saw firsthand how physical activity kept my grandmother independent and living in her own home until the last month of her life. Her sister Liz, on the other hand, spent years in a long-term care facility, wasting away. Liz was much more sedentary than her sisters. My grandmother had an active life taking care of her husband and home, and my other great-aunt, Addie, was a regular at her building's indoor pool well into her eighties. I always remember that my Auntie Liz seemed to disappear into the couch — she spent a lot of time sitting and she struck me for many years as being frail beyond her years.

Looking back, I often wonder if I could have helped her be more active. Would it have helped if I had encouraged her to go for a walk when I visited? I'll never know for sure. But in my practice as a fitness professional, I see women and men who remind me of Auntie Liz. They may have joined one of my fitness classes earlier in their retirement years or hired me as a personal trainer to visit their home. A few of them bought workout handbooks and exercise DVDs geared to seniors, but they often found them too difficult to follow. Here are some of the reasons I heard:

- They can't or won't get on the floor to work out.
- They don't have the equipment for the workouts and they're not willing to buy it.
- They can't stand for long periods and would like some seated exercise options.
- They don't know how to do the exercises safely, in some cases because the exercises are too advanced and they need a simplified version.

I know that some seniors might never step foot in a gym. Does this sound like you? The gym isn't for everyone, and that's okay. But exercise still matters, and mobile personal trainers like me offer hope for seniors like you to remain independent. I take this role very seriously. I hope this book will help you stay mobile and independent — and upright — for as long as possible. Like I said earlier, we all have a "physical" best-before date, and I want the best for you before your body hits that date.

PART ONE: THE PROBLEM

FEAR OF FALLING

Sphinx: "What creature goes on four feet in the morning, two at noonday, and three in the evening?"
Oedipus: "Man."
— *Sophocles (429 BC)*[1]

Is Fear a Vicious Circle?

Fear of falling keeps some people from getting up and moving more. Does this feel familiar? Unfortunately, lack of movement further weakens our muscles, stiffens our joints, and reduces our ability to balance. I've seen it many times: A senior has a fall and injures themselves. As they recover from their injury, they become less mobile and sure-footed, so they move less. Then the movement feels forced and unnatural, which further saps their confidence, so they move even less. Then their bodies become weaker, stiffer, and more unbalanced, so they move less still.

Can you relate to this scenario? A single fall can undermine your confidence and impact your activity level. Thus begins the vicious cycle of falls. With this book, I want to build your confidence. I want to show you that there are safe ways to strengthen your body and improve your balance. It's what I do with my senior clients during fitness house calls.

Have You Ever Fallen?

Have you ever fallen? I have fallen more than once, but one fall in particular stands out in my head. It was a dark winter evening, and the walking conditions were less than ideal. I was heading out back to our car. Just as I passed the garage, I slipped on the ice and fell. Try as I might, I couldn't stand up on the slippery driveway.

Even though I was only about 30 feet from our back door, I knew I needed help. I pulled out my cell phone and called our home phone.

"I've fallen and I can't get up." Sound familiar? It reminded me of a television commercial I first saw as a child. You might remember it too. In it, an older, grey-haired woman uttered the phrase from her bathroom floor. While I may have had some grey hairs peeking around the edges, I was only 43 years old when I said it.

As I waited for my kids to come to my rescue — they arrived quite quickly, actually, but still lovingly tease me about it to this day — I thought of how many seniors fall at home, just like in the commercial. And they don't always have someone who can help them.

As a fitness professional, I realized that I could help seniors take charge of their lives and reduce their risk of falling. While you'll need to consult with Mother Nature and municipal road crews about the state of icy sidewalks in the winter, I can help you improve your balance, strength, and mobility to decrease the likelihood of falling both in your home and when you're out and about — ice and snow being the exception, of course. Exercise works wonders to help you avoid a fall.

What's the Problem with Falling?

As we age, our risk of falling increases, as does the likelihood that a fall will cause an injury. In Canada, falls are the leading cause of injury among older Canadians. Twenty to thirty percent of seniors experience one or more falls each year. Falls are the cause of 85 percent of seniors' injury-related hospitalizations. You may be surprised to learn that falls are the cause of 95 percent of all hip fractures and fully half of all falls causing hospitalization happen at home.[2]

In the United States, data reported by the National Council on Aging show that one quarter of Americans over the age of 65 will fall each year. Falls are also the prevailing reason for hospital admissions among the elderly. An emergency room in the United States treats a senior fall victim every 11 seconds. And if you're an older adult, you're more likely to die from a fall than any other cause.[3]

In the past, research attributed the risk of falls exclusively to aging. That is to say, the likelihood of a fall was simply connected to the year we were born. In fact, it's more like aging and lack of physical activity are working together to increase the likelihood that we will fall. As we age, we are typically less active. Our bodies get weaker, our bones get more brittle, and that is why we're more likely to fall. And when we do suffer a fall later in life, we're also more likely to be injured.

Researcher and professor Robert Wood is featured in a YouTube video called "Why Seniors Fall."[4] In the video, Wood offers simple tips for exercises that can be incorporated into your daily routine, such as drawing the letters of the alphabet with your foot. This helps increase flexibility in your ankle and strengthen the muscles up your shin, which are both important to help you lift your foot as you walk, and thus prevent a fall. My mother was the one who first alerted me to Dr. Wood's terrific video because, as she said, "It's just like all the exercises you have us do in your exercise class."

She was right. Dr. Wood's video demonstrated fundamental exercises that equip seniors with muscular strength and good balance. I focus on similar skills in my exercise classes and one-on-one sessions with seniors.

EXERCISE VS. GETTING IN SHAPE

*"It is exercise alone that supports the spirits,
and keeps the mind in vigor."*
— *Cicero (106-43 BC)*

Are You in Shape?

What does it mean to be in shape? The answer is, "It depends." Everyone has different fitness goals, and our opinion of whether or not we're in shape relates directly to those goals. Another way to think about it is this: Do you live to exercise or exercise to live? For me, I want to live a long and healthy life, so I exercise for life. I also exercise for disease prevention because exercise IS medicine.

For many of my clients, their fitness goals relate to the "exercising to live" side of the coin. For example, I hear things like:

- "I'm scared I'm going to fall again."

- "I've been very unsteady and unsure of my footing."
- "I haven't fully recovered from my surgery."
- "I want to get stronger before my hip replacement surgery."
- "I know I should get on the floor to exercise, but I'm embarrassed about how difficult it is for me to get down and back up."
- "I want to be able to pick up my two-year-old grandson when he runs up to me."

So you see, being in shape means different things to different people based on their uniquely personal fitness goals. And so they exercise. If all of our muscles are strong and responsive, they're all fulfilling their intended roles, and we operate like a finely tuned machine. If there's a muscular imbalance, our bones get pulled closer together, causing joint pain and postural misalignment. Other muscles have to pick up the slack and our entire system gets out of whack. Consider an assembly line where one worker isn't pulling their weight: other workers have to double their efforts until they reach a breaking point and the system falls apart.

But how much *should* we exercise as we age? Let me shed some light on that question by sharing the physical activity recommendations.

How Much and What Type of Exercise Do You Need?

The Canadian Physical Activity Guidelines recommend that adults engage in 150 minutes of moderate to vigorous physical activity every week to maintain optimal health. The guidelines also recommend that we do strength training two days per week to maintain our muscles and bones.[5] The guidelines for Canadians over the age of 65 also include a recommendation for balance exercises where needed.[6] I would argue that anyone over the age of 40 should be thinking about — and even doing — balance exercises on a regular basis. As I get ready to enter my 50s, I do all the same balance exercises that I teach my senior clients. They help me, and they can help you too.

The American Physical Activity Guidelines are almost identical to the Canadian recommendations.[7] That's because many countries have been revising their physical activity guidelines to present a united front to their citizens.[8] It doesn't matter where you live, physical activity is important for your overall health.

While I would love for all of my clients to complete 150 minutes of physical activity every week, I recognize that for many people, this is unlikely. I see it in the types of fitness goals my senior clients identify, including some of the examples I listed in the last section, and I understand that vigorous physical activity may be *too much* vigor for some seniors. And that's okay, because as we age, we tend to slow down and do less. According to Professor Wood, "the person that has not been active has the most to gain by becoming active."[9] Every minute of movement counts, especially that first one.[10]

Walking is the preferred form of exercise for many adults of all ages. I love to walk too. Unless you have specific mobility challenges, walking is a simple and free form of physical activity. Your steps can be recorded using a pedometer, accelerometer, or an app that often comes with modern smart phones, and many adults I know subscribe to the general recommendation of accumulating 10,000 steps per day to maintain your health.

However, some older adults may need a nudge to accumulate those steps. A Canadian research study that used accelerometers to track physical activity found that adults aged 60 to 79 recorded significantly lower step counts than their younger counterparts — 7,000 to 7,900 steps per day for the seniors versus 8,700 to 10,000 steps per day for those aged 20 to 59.[11]

And, as I mentioned earlier, reduced activity can further increase the chances of an injury-inducing fall. Even if you're already participating in a walking pro-

gram, you can still benefit from the exercises in this book. When it comes to reducing your risk of falling, you need to work on balance, strength, and mobility.[12] Some of the questions I often ask clients — and that I invite you to ask yourself — are:
- "Can you cross the street before the traffic light changes?"
- "Can you lift your foot high enough to clear a step?"
- "Can you get in and out of a chair without help?"

If you said no to one or more of these questions, I am here to help you. Together, we can work on increasing your light physical activity levels using the exercises in this book, which you can easily learn to do at home.

Are There Benefits to Light Physical Activity?

Recently, an image was circulating online that depicts the extremes of aging. There were side-by-side photos of two 80-year-old women; one of them was stooped over a walker and the other was flexing her muscles at a bodybuilding competition. The caption asked readers to ponder which way they wanted to age.

My first thought was that binary options — yes or no, on or off — presented in categories that represent a continuum can be problematic and inaccurate. I appreciate the attention-grabbing visual that polar opposites represent, but they don't tell the whole story, and I worry that these extreme comparisons will discourage the thousands of seniors whose reality lies somewhere between these distant boundaries.

Physical activity lies on a continuum. Fitness professionals use tools such as the Rating of Perceived Exertion (RPE) Scale to subjectively measure how hard we're working during exercise.[13] With the RPE Scale, you rate how you feel on a scale of one to ten — a concept that most people can quickly grasp. On the low end of the scale, one represents low activity: minimal exertion and the ability to talk and breathe normally, like standing. On the high end of the scale, ten represents maximum intensity: the high-performance zone, "severe" exertion and gasping for breath, like you're in a race that you're trying to win.

Most of my clients are working towards the lower end of the scale, in what's referred to as the health improvement zone. Research suggests that this kind of light physical activity is as beneficial to older adults and sedentary individuals as more vigorous exercise is for younger and more physically fit Canadians.[14]

BALANCE AND GRAVITY

"There is more to life than increasing its speed."
— Gandhi

How's Your Balance?

Think about your current health. How's your balance? Can you close your eyes whilst standing on one leg? If so, can you hold that pose for 15 to 30 seconds? Most adults don't even realize their balance has deteriorated until after they fall and hurt themselves. And let me tell you, falling is not age-specific. However, as we age, our chances of experiencing a fall increase drastically. And as we discussed earlier, you're more likely to be injured from a fall the older you are.

We all need good balance to safely move around our world on a daily basis, but it's easy to take it for granted. If you've ever lost your balance, fallen, and sustained an injury, you get it. Balance is a critical component of walking, which is basically just a process of transferring our weight from side to side and maintaining an upright posture. With each step, we shift our weight from one foot to the other. If you have trouble with balance, then it makes sense that you would also have trouble walking. And it's when you're walking that you're most likely to fall.

If balance is a challenge for you, you're likely more aware of the importance of being able to maintain an upright position without falling over. It's cute when a toddler is learning to walk and they tip over. A young child falls regularly, but over time, their balance improves and they fall less often. As adults age, poor balance can be life-threatening and, quite frankly, frightening.

Whether we like it or not, as we get older, our balance is negatively impacted by our aging bodies. Let's take a closer look at what our bodies are going through:

- Cells die in our vestibular system, which is connected to the part of our brain that controls balance.
- Our vision declines and with it, our depth perception.
- Changes to our blood pressure may cause dizziness, light-headedness or blurriness.

- We lose muscle mass, strength, and power, which can slow our reaction time if we trip.
- Our reflexes and coordination decline.
- A variety of health problems can impact our balance, including arthritis, stroke, Parkinson's disease and multiple sclerosis.[15]

Regular physical activity is the key to maintaining good balance. An exercise program that focuses on specific balance exercises as well as core strengthening and movement patterns will improve balance and stability, not to mention daily function. The exercises in this book are geared to helping you avoid a fall. I hope you'll see that exercise does not need to be complicated.

Do You Know about the Heel-Toe Express?

As I mentioned earlier, walking is the main form of physical activity for many older adults. It's a great low-cost, uncomplicated way to stay active. And proper walking form can achieve all of the fitness goals that will help prevent a slip, trip, or fall.

As we discussed in last section, walking is essentially a dynamic balance exercise: you constantly shift your weight from one foot to the other and back again. To successfully accomplish this dynamic balance work, your muscles need to be strong enough to continuously lift your feet and clear the ground safely. Your bones and muscles in your torso must be strong enough to maintain an upright posture. And your balance is being continuously challenged as you shift your centre of gravity and base of support (more on those concepts later).

Ironically, though, walking is when most falls occur because one or more of these components is coming up short. But there's an easy fix, and if you keep reading I'll show you.

What's Gravity Got to Do With It?

What do astronauts on the International Space Station have in common with someone who is bedridden with an illness or injury? It's not a trick question. The answer is "no gravity." Being horizontal for extended periods of time impacts bodily functions, so much so that NASA paid test subjects $18,000 to lie in bed for 70 days while being poked, prodded, and monitored.[16] Then they asked them to try standing up for 15 minutes. It sounds easy enough, but it wasn't.

Our bodies don't like to be sedentary for very long. After a while, our organs and systems start to decay. This can include decreased blood volume, reduced bone density, loss of muscle strength, disappearance of fine and gross motor skills, and vanishing balance and mobility. Our hearts have to pump harder to move blood throughout our bodies, bed sores can develop on our skin, and our emotional well-being also takes a hit.[17]

The NASA study was an effort to assess the physiological impact of extended space travel to Mars, but, as with many NASA initiatives, the results have real-world implications on Earth right now. How can older adults with physical limitations and mobility issues maintain independence while fighting the effects of zero-gravity from extended bed time?

Mobility is critical for maintaining independence and for keeping costly, long-term care services to a minimum. According to researchers in the United States, a six-month delay in entering a nursing home can reduce health care costs by millions.[18] These same researchers are working to identify older adults who are at risk of disability and creating customized exercise programs to prevent an inevitable downward slide. And guess what they're focusing on in terms of activity? The strength and balance required to lift one foot after the other, whether it's to climb the stairs or to simply walk *to* those stairs.

Here's how one of the NASA research participants described his first walk after 70 days in bed: "With a staff member on each side...I sat up on the stretcher and stepped down onto the ground. My feet tingled like they were sluggish and short as I dragged my feet across the ground and kicked my ankles. I lacked all the fine coordination skills that I hadn't used for months. I felt sharp pains in my ankles and feet as I pivoted through the obstacle course, and I certainly couldn't walk a straight line well." It didn't last, though: "Within a few days of casual strolling and formal reconditioning exercise, my balance returned and my endurance began to recover."[19]

Bottom line, if you experience an extended period of time in a horizontal position — bed-ridden — please make an effort to get out of bed and let gravity work on your body. You can do this by standing next to your bed before you begin moving. Then, you can slowly increase movement and activity every day. It's not too late, and your body will thank you for it. Not sure how to start? We'll cover the basics and more in the next section.

PART TWO:
THE SOLUTION

FALL PREVENTION

"The doctor of the future will give no medicine, but instead will interest his patients in the care of the human frame, in diet, and in the cause and prevention of disease."
— Thomas Edison

Want to Hear About My First Encounter with Fall Prevention?

I completed graduate school in 1993. Soon after, I joined the local health department's Community Health Research Unit, and fall prevention among seniors was one of my first project assignments.

"How do you prevent seniors from falling?" I asked the project coordinator shortly after joining the team. Although my elderly grandparents and two great-aunts had featured prominently in my childhood, none of them had experienced a life-altering fall. So in my youthful naivety, the idea of a research project to prevent falls seemed a bit far-fetched.

Her response was an eye-opener to me: "We conduct in-home assessments, where we coach seniors to not walk around in slippery stockings or socks, to keep bathroom floors dry, reduce clutter in the home, improve lighting, and remove or secure slippery area rugs."

To be honest, I don't recall if there was a physical activity component to the project. At the time, the thought didn't even cross my mind. It was much later when I began thinking about it — the importance of equipping older adults to be strong and balanced. Last year, I picked up a flyer at our local hospital and started thinking about the topic even more.

Have You Seen Fall Prevention Programs Lately?

The flyer was called "How to reduce your fall risk at home."[20] In addition to environmental adjustments like the ones mentioned above, it also emphasized physical fitness. The fitness components resonated with me because they focused on bone and muscle strength as well as balance. These factors are critical to staying strong and upright — that is, avoiding falls. In fact, the flyer highlighted that exercise and physical activity are the best way to nip those nose dives in the bud. I couldn't agree more.

Although exercise was listed as the most important factor, the tips on *how* to get more exercise was the shortest section. The flyer rightly recommended that individuals contact their doctor before beginning an exercise program. In the fitness world, many of us use tools like the PAR-Q (Physical Activity Readiness Questionnaire) to assess readiness to exercise.[21] And I have actually sent prospective clients back to their physician for follow-up before I've agreed to take them on as personal training clients or accepted them into my seniors' fitness classes.

Unfortunately, many individuals mistakenly expect their physician to develop an exercise plan. I've had potential clients contact me and say things like, "My doctor told me I need to exercise more but not what kind of exercise I should do." And that's okay, because that's where people like me come in. I love helping people figure out what is going to work for them.

Can You Regain Your Confidence after a Fall?

I visit private homes, community centres, and retirement homes to help seniors get more active. Every group and every individual is different, and yet I see the same issues cropping up again and again. People need strong muscles and bones to walk unaided, and they need to work on their balance so that if they do experience a slip or trip, they'll be able to catch themselves before they fall. Finally, they need to rebuild their confidence to keep moving.

After I fell on the ice, it took me a few days to feel comfortable walking outside in poor conditions again. But then I realized that I needed to take charge of my health and prepare myself to get back outside. Before long, I was back to walking — slowly and with control — on icy surfaces. My clients also tell me they feel more confident after we work together. One of them even accepted an invitation to go walking immediately following her workout with me, something she told me she wouldn't have done previously.

The following chapters will describe the fundamental fitness components for fall prevention. Then, the Action Plan will provide guidance on how you can do these exercises at home.

BALANCE BASICS

"Self-care is never a selfish act — it is simply good stewardship of the only gift I have."
— Parker Palmer

Do You Know the Three Pillars of Balance?

Our balance system is complex and relies on sensory input from three distinct systems: visual, vestibular, and proprioceptive (also known as somatosensory). All of this is just a fancy way of describing how our bodies process information.[22] Let me break them down.

Visual system: As you might guess, this is about our eyes, which provide visual input to our brains as we move through life.

Vestibular system: This is the medical term for the inner ear, which processes sensory information about motion, equilibrium, and spatial orientation. Close your eyes and slowly move your head side to side. Your vestibular system is now sending crucial input to your brain. As we age, our side-to-side head movements become less frequent, which negatively impacts our vestibular system. In other words, it doesn't work if we don't use it. "Use it or lose it" doesn't just apply to our muscles — it applies to every single part of our bodies.

Proprioception or somatosensory: This is our brain's ability to sense our body's position in space. That's why we can walk through our house in the dark without falling down, unless of course, we bang into an unseen object. The nerves in our body send signals to our brain that allow us to maintain an upright position, and we have just as many sensors (i.e., nerve endings) in the bottom of our feet as we do in our entire spinal column. That's why it's so important to remove our shoes every day and activate those sensors on the bottoms of our feet. Also, the nerve endings in our spinal column rely on posture to determine our body's orientation as it moves. That's why posture is a key component of balance and preventing falls.

Is It a Photo or a Video?

Balance is a "sweet spot" between our base of support — typically our feet — and our centre of gravity — our weight distribution — while we're moving or standing still in an upright position. As we move through life, the dynamic aspect is key. We are creatures of movement, and most people want to continue to move. But our aging bodies sometimes have difficulty balancing the key balance components (pun intended). Our balance can suffer as we become less mobile.

Imagine a dog walking on a slippery surface. They appear more sure-footed than their human counterparts, who are often slip-sliding along the ice. That's because the dogs have a lower centre of gravity and a wider base of support.

Static balance involves maintaining your centre of gravity over your base of support. I like to compare the practice of standing upright to a still photograph. Dynamic balance is when your centre of gravity moves away from your base of support, but you are still in control. That is, your muscles are firing to keep you from falling to the ground. That's when your balance is more like a video.

The exercises in this book target both static and dynamic balance because they're both important and need to be maintained.

Can You Improve Your Balance in Three Days?

You don't have to be older to be concerned about your balance. We all need good balance to safely move around on a daily basis, but have you ever thought much about it? As we age, poor balance can lead to injury.

As part of The Move More Institute™, I created several online courses to help clients improve their balance. The first course, called "Three Days to Better Balance," was designed to improve body awareness, strengthen the brain-body connection, and learn how to engage more muscles during simple everyday activities like standing and walking.

The second course, called "Balance 2.0: Progressions in Motion," teaches participants how to control their body's position in motion and improve their coordination. It also teaches them how to walk sideways — to strengthen the smaller muscles on the sides of the legs — and how to use core muscle strength when moving.

Initially, I asked participants if they could foresee any barriers to successfully completing the courses.

That is, what would stand in the way of improving their balance during either of the three-day courses. Responses included: self-doubt, no social support, sticking to a schedule, motivation, and consistency.

During the course, I checked in with them every day to encourage and support their progress and provide expertise. Based on feedback after the course, participants appreciated the extra support. They told me it helped improve their self-confidence and preserve their motivation to continue. They also shared that the course increased their awareness of the factors impacting balance and the habits they needed to integrate into daily life.

Here's what some of them said:
- "I became very aware of my standing base when I stood at the sink doing my teeth or stood at the bus stop."
- "Wow, so great for my unconscious winter hunched shoulders' posture!"
- "I really needed the 3-Day Balance work. It was great."

I share these comments to show you that I can help you even though we're not working together in real time. The guidance I provide in this book can be used over and over, as you learn and perfect the exercises I recommend. One of the most basic exercises you'll learn is how to activate your body when you walk.

How's Your Walking?

Walking is an exercise in dynamic balancing. Steady yourself on one foot, then the other. Repeat. If you're already having trouble with static balance, how will your body respond to walking? Well, walking will also be difficult, and that's when you're most likely to risk a fall. Can you sustain repeated shifts in your centre of gravity and base of support as you move forward? Are your legs strong enough to lift those feet off the ground without catching your big toe? And you don't need to have grey hair to be concerned about falling whilst walking. That's why I love this quote about the power of walking for all ages:

"*So Many Reasons to Walk.* Walking is our original exercise. You have been doing it since you were a baby. Of all activities, walking may just be the safest, simplest, most social, spiritual and brain activating. Walking strengthens the bones, heart, core muscles and legs…walking is great in all stages of life, from childhood on through your middle and senior years."[23]

We'll revisit the mechanics of walking in the next section. For now, let's see how my course participants fared with the guidelines on how to change their walking style:

"It is a bit strange; it seemed unnatural doing it around the house. But this morning I was out snowshoeing and when I paid attention, it was very natural. I just watched the video again and this time it was better."

"I had to watch [the video] three times before I could walk deliberately and not feel that I was off-balance…I will definitely practice more tonight."

These comments reflect what happens in our bodies and brains as we deliberately try to change how we move and re-learn the mechanics of walking. Our brains think our "off-balanced" way of walking is normal, so when we make corrections, the old grey matter — that's the grey inside our heads, not on them — is worried that we're actually off-balance. It takes some time to master because we are retraining both our muscles and our brains.

BALANCE AND STRENGTH

"If a man achieves victory over this body, who in the world can exercise power over him? He who rules himself rules over the whole world."
— *Vinoba Bhave*

Have You Ever Tripped Over Your Own Foot?

Strong muscles and bones allow us to lift our legs and feet over obstacles like pesky snow piles that haven't been cleared. Or our big toe. When the muscles in our legs are weak, it's more difficult to lift our feet off the ground as we walk. When that happens, our own body becomes a trip hazard.

It comes back to the importance of using our muscles to keep them functioning and strong. It means the difference between maintaining our independence or requiring help with daily activities. Our bodies need to be strong in both static and dynamic poses. When we walk, the leg on the ground and our entire torso need to hold us upright and our moving leg must be strong enough to clear obstacles, including that pesky toe.

If you're reading this book, I'm going to assume you want to maintain your independence by keeping your body strong.

What Does It Mean to Exercise?

What does it mean to exercise? Do you need to be able to power lift a heavy barbell? Or can it simply be that you're strong enough to independently complete your activities of daily living? And how does that independence relate to physical activity?

The World Health Organization defines physical activity as "any bodily movement produced by skeletal muscles that requires energy expenditure."[24] I don't see anything in that definition that mentions sweating, special clothing, "feeling the burn," or a gym membership. It tells us that movement — any movement — is physical activity and will benefit your body.

For example, if you do your own housework, you're already doing physical activity. That counts as exercise in my book. Let me break it down for you.

Vacuuming: You're pushing, pulling, and lifting. If you have a two-storey house, you carry the beastly machine up and down the stairs. It's all added weight that you're moving around, along with your own body weight. That's a form of strength training.

Dusting or washing windows: You stretch and reach away from your centre of gravity. You pull your muscles into an elongated position and either hold them there or move in this stretched-out position. That, my friend, qualifies as dynamic balance and flexibility training.

Washing the floor: You vigorously wash away stains and get your heart pumping. There's even a bead of sweat on your brow. You just completed cardiovascular training — aka, vigorous physical activity.

So embrace your chores — they help you increase your activity level, keeping your muscles and bones strong. For free. And even if you have help with your housework, you can still be physically active in your home. Take the stairs, for example. I'm not being disrespectful, I really want you to climb those stairs.

Will Those Stairs Really Kill You?

I live in an older neighbourhood with tall, narrow infill developments. Large, stately, old brick homes butt up against three- and four-storey townhomes. It's a desirable neighbourhood for many age groups, young and old alike. Young families will share a wall with retirees who left the suburbs for a smaller footprint in a walkable neighbourhood.

In one of these vertical townhouse developments, a widowed grandmother in her 80s moved in, much to the chagrin of her adult children. "There are too many stairs in that house. They're going to kill you!" To which she replied, "Are you kidding? These stairs are going to keep me alive. Every time I go up and down, I'm getting stronger and I'm maintaining good balance. If I lived in a one-level apartment or a bungalow, my muscles would disappear from disuse!"

And she's right. Climbing stairs in our home is a fantastic — and free — way to maintain lower body strength and balance. Just like walking, climbing stairs is a dynamic balance act that requires us to constantly shift our centre of gravity from one foot to the other. Our heart pumps from the added exertion, so we can tick "cardio workout" off our to-do list. We load our bones against gravity as we climb, not to mention the strength required in our muscles to continually lift one foot after the other to the next step.

Can You Do a Side Shuffle?

Strength matters to all of our muscles, not just the ones that propel us forward or upwards. Take sideways walking, for example.

Sideways walking strengthens the little-used muscles along the inside and outside of our legs, which can help improve balance. And it's great brain training, too. Since we don't typically walk sideways, our body and brain have to exert more effort to move. This new movement creates new pathways in our brain because our body has to rely on messages the nerves in our feet are sending to the penthouse. Additionally, sideways walking improves coordination in our lower body.

I hope I've convinced you that good balance requires a strong body. Another aspect of keeping our body strong is our posture, which we'll examine next.

BALANCE AND POSTURE

"We are born with every muscle, bone and joint we need to move in a fluid, deliberate and healthy way."
— Mel Fiala, athletic therapist

How Does Your Posture Impact Your Fall Risk?

When you have a stooped posture — whether it's due to weak muscles, too much sitting, or years of slouching forward at a desk — your centre of gravity is no longer over your base of support. In this case, if you catch your foot on something and slip, momentum will propel you forward. And it's very difficult to pull yourself back and up once momentum takes over.

In this hunched-over position, your bones are not aligned, and you can't support your body weight. Instead, your muscles and your connective tissue — the tendons that connect muscles to bones and ligaments that connect bones to each other — have been assigned a role that's normally reserved for your bones. Eventually, these muscles, tendons, and ligaments declare a strike because they already have a job to do. They don't want a second job. It's like asking the widget makers to also make sprockets; they'd rather stick to making widgets and let the sprocket makers make the sprockets.

Think of your body as a finely-tuned, highly specialized assembly line. Every part of our body is designed for its specialty. If you don't use all the parts in the right way, they'll stop functioning. In the case of movement, if you're going to keep moving, other parts will have to jump in and help. And that's when you risk falling.

It's not too late to start. Your body has an incredible feedback loop of action-reaction. If you begin to work your muscles and load your bones, your body will respond. But if you don't use them, you will lose them.

Do You Play the Piano?

A *long* time ago, when I was in seventh grade, my teacher commented on how good a fellow student's posture was. Even though most of us were bored with the lesson, this student was sitting completely upright. The rest of us were either slumped over our desks with our eyes just inches from our worksheet or leaning against the chair's backrest.

The teacher continued to praise her and exclaimed, "You must take piano lessons! I can tell someone has drilled into you the importance of good posture." I guiltily sat upright at that point; my organ teacher was regularly chastising me for slouching during our lessons.

Your piano (or organ) teacher was right. Or maybe it was your mother who told you to sit up straight. If you are holding your body upright instead of relying on furniture, your muscles are working. Many of us outsource the job of our muscles to our chairs when we constantly slouch instead of sitting more actively.

How do you sit in a chair? Do you make your muscles hold you in an upright position, or have you outsourced their role to the furniture by slumping backwards?

To sit actively, we need to load our muscles and bones to fight the effects of gravity, and we must avoid outsourcing the role of our muscles by slumping in our seats. If you're hunched forward in your upper spine, your lower spine is probably tucked under, causing painful and unnecessary loading of the muscles, tendons, and ligaments.

Learning how to sit actively will engage muscles and load bones. It will improve posture, breathing, and mood, and it will make you stronger. Imagine that: sitting as a form of exercise. At the end of one fitness house call, my client Cynthia said to me, "It's amazing you can still work your body in a chair. I feel wonderful."

Do You Window Shop?

Do you check your reflection when you are window shopping? I don't mean standing in front a mirror and checking your posture. I mean when you're out and about, not thinking about your posture. That's the best time to check what I call your natural posture — how you actually hold yourself when you're not conscious of it.

I try to check my reflection every few months. The first time I did this many years ago, I was shocked at what I saw. My shoulders were slouched forward and I looked much shorter than I actually am. It made me think of the fallacy that everyone shrinks as they age. It's not that we're actually getting shorter, we're just no longer using our bodies the way they were meant to be used. There's no good reason for losing height. If you work on your posture, muscle strength, and joint mobility, you will remain the same height throughout your adult years.

I teach my clients how to stand actively, so they can simultaneously improve their balance and posture. Not sure what active standing means? Let me explain.

Are You a Comma, Question Mark, or Exclamation Point?

Think about yourself again for a moment. When you stand, does your body look like a comma, a question mark, or an exclamation point? Hint: the latter is the preferred position. It takes about 100 muscles working together in your body to maintain good posture and correct alignment. Standing actively is a static balance exercise, with your centre of gravity positioned over your base of support in a "freeze mode." It's also a strength activity in which your muscles and bones are fully engaged in maintaining your skeleton in an upright position. Good balance and posture are inextricably linked; you can't have one without the other.

The goal with active standing is to align our bones and the weight-bearing joints of our body. They're the parts of our body that are meant to support us, not our muscles, tendons, and ligaments. When our joints are out of alignment, we have to rely on connective tissue like tendons and ligaments to hold us upright. This practice causes wear and tear on the joints, unnecessary strain on the connective tissue, and it weakens the bones that are not being loaded with our body weight. Not only can it lead to pain and discomfort, but it can also increase your risk of falling.

Wear and tear on our joints is the topic of the next chapter, and I'll explain how lack of movement degrades them.

BALANCE AND YOUR JOINTS

> *"In our daily lives, many of us forget that we have a body. Our bodies often contain stress, pain, and suffering. Often we ignore the body until the pain gets too great."*
> — Thich Nhat Hanh

Are Your Ankles Stiff?

Our bodies are brilliant machines that are designed to move — all day, every day. In our daily lives, we twist, we turn, we bend, we reach, and we lift. We use our bodies as a unit, and we expect to be able to move every which way without pain or having to worry about proper alignment.

If all of our muscles are strong and our joints are mobile, they're all fulfilling their intended roles and we operate like a finely-tuned machine. If there's a muscular imbalance, bones get pulled closer together, causing joint pain and postural misalignment.

When I run workshops for office workers, I often have participants try to walk around with "stiff" ankles. I instruct them to lock their ankles so they can't flex their feet as they take each step. Then I ask them how it makes the rest of their body feel. How quickly do you think you can walk with stiff ankles? When our feet and ankles are immobile, it can affect our balance, posture, and walking speed. When I work with seniors who are less mobile, this lesson becomes moot. For the most part, they're already walking with stiff ankles, so they don't need to be convinced that this immobility needs to be addressed.

Are You a Well-Oiled Machine?

When you move, do you feel as stiff as a robot? Does the feeling fade over time? If it fades, that's a good sign because the movement you're doing is helping to lubricate your joints. I'm here to tell you that you need to do more of it.

Joints are the connections between our bones, where two or more bones meet. Our muscles pull our bones towards or away from joints, depending on the movement we're doing. Spoiler alert: our muscles do all the work, and our bones and joints are just along for the ride. But when those joints aren't being used, such as when we're less active, the joints dry up.

If you're feeling particularly stiff and creaky one day and you have to speed up — for instance, if you're crossing the street and the light changes midway through your curb-to-curb excursion — stiff joints will make it difficult for you to act quickly. Your body may feel like a robot trying to ride a bicycle. Although the parts are moving, it looks forced and unnatural, and your reaction time is slower when those joints are rigid and dry. This rigidity and slower feedback between your body and your brain put you at greater risk of a fall.

But there's an easy fix. Has a health or fitness professional ever told you that motion is lotion? Or that movement is medicine? I'm guilty of using those phrases because they are effective ways to remind people that their bodies — including their joints — need and crave movement. And slow-motion, circular movements are the key to this lock.[25]

Do You Play with CARs?

My philosophy is the slower the movement, the better. Large rotations and circles performed s-l-o-w-l-y to follow all the possible angles at which each joint can move. And there's a great acronym to help you remember what you need to do: CARs. I'll let certified athletic trainer Cassandra McCoy explain them:

"CARs means Controlled Articular Rotations. As you do the exercise, you are making controlled movements within each joint articulation against gravity via a big rotation. The best thing is the more that you do them, the stronger you get, and the bigger your circle will become. You can start out with a baby circle working within your current range and then gradually, as you get stronger, that range of motion will get bigger."[26]

Having a limited range of motion in our joints can cause fear, because we're worried what will happen *if* we have to move quickly. So the key is to increase the range of our joints slowly, to allay our fears and increase our confidence. With CARs, we draw bigger and bigger circles in a controlled manner. Circles are 360 degrees; we have 360 joints in our body. And with all this talk of circles, it's time for me to tell you we've come full circle with our discussion of balance, strength, and mobility. Now it's time to move on to the action of improving balance.

PART THREE:
THE ACTION PLAN

FUNCTIONAL FITNESS

*"There is no such thing as perfect movement,
but there is always better movement."*
— Moshé Feldenkrais

Does Practice Make Perfect?

No doubt you've heard the saying "practice makes perfect." You may have even uttered those words yourself. I know I have in the past, but not anymore. Instead, I now focus on progress over perfection. With the bulk of my private clients over the age of 70, we celebrate small wins and progress, and we leave the pursuit of perfection to the younger folks. As I mentioned earlier, these are some of the fitness goals I work on with these clients:

- "I want to be able to go for a walk with my husband."
- "I want to get stronger before my surgery."

- "I don't want to fall and hurt myself."
- "I want to have the energy to play with my grandchildren."

You get the idea — practice makes progress. And that's why I focus on functional fitness with my clients.

What's Functional Fitness?

Have you ever heard the term "functional fitness?" It refers to exercises that help train our body to do everyday activities with ease and without pain. For example, a squat is functional because it's training the act of sit-to-stand (or the opposite, stand-to-sit) — a movement we do dozens of times every single day. It also allows us to be in control of our body as we lower ourselves to — and lift ourselves from — a seat, whether it's a recliner, a toilet, or your car.

It can be as simple as not wanting to fall when dropping onto the sofa. My mother-in-law told me that she loves sinking into her comfy chair when she's tired and wants to sit down. She's letting gravity take hold instead of using her muscles to lower her body with control. I asked her to imagine what would happen if she did the same thing to sit on the toilet. She agreed that it might cause her to hurt her back. And that's where functional fitness comes in.

Functional fitness increases strength, trains muscles to work together, improves balance, and reduces the risk of a fall. I ask my clients to think about that next time they sit down in a comfy recliner. Then I ask them to slow down the movement and take control of their body, to not outsource the job of their muscles to gravity. Can you relate? The exercises in the next chapter will help you retain control of your body as you go about your day.

Do You Know How to Turn a Movement into Exercise?

In my last book, I advocated for adopting non-exercise activity to counteract the harmful effects of a sedentary lifestyle — moving your body more to improve your health and well-being.[27] In this book, I describe specific movements that I want you to do on a daily basis. Basically, I show you how to turn a movement into an exercise.

For example, you sit down many times every single day. If I tell you to take one of those moments and repeat the movement five times, that's an exercise. Stand up. Sit down. Stand up. Sit down. Stand up. Sit down. These repetitions are now considered exercise.

It's that easy to add a little exercise to your day. As you work through the exercises, you can begin doing them as single movements — try it on for size, so to speak. Once you're comfortable, repeat the movement to boost your balance, increase your strength, and enhance your joint mobility.

Can We Talk About Safety?

Before we proceed, let's talk about safety. As with other fitness texts, my book includes a disclaimer in the front: "The information in this book should not be used for diagnosis or treatment, or as a substitute for professional medical care. Before beginning any exercise program, consult your physician." That's not just legal jargon for the sake of it, it's important advice to heed because everyone's health is different.

But there's more: I want you to use your common sense. The tips in this book are meant to help you, not hurt you. If something bothers you, stop doing it. The balance exercises are meant to improve your balance, not make you fall down. Always make sure you have something sturdy to hang onto — a counter, a wall, a chair that won't slip, or a fellow human, be it a relative, a friend, or a personal trainer.

If you have any questions at all about the exercises listed here, take this book to your doctor or other health professional and review it with them. Or you can hire a personal trainer in your neighbourhood to work with you. There are many great fitness professionals who work with older adults just like you.

And remember, the goal is to make you stronger and improve your balance. Even small increments of activity and exercise will get you closer to this goal. Shall we get started?

THE EXERCISES

"Exercise? I thought you said 'extra fries'!"
— Anonymous (Unknown)

Tackling the Exercises One at a Time

Finding time to do these exercises doesn't have to be complicated. When I work with clients in their homes, I send follow-up emails that list and describe the exercises we've done together. My goal is to make clients comfortable doing the exercises on their own. In many cases, they write out the exercises on a sheet of paper for quick reference. You know, something that they can leave on the counter and refer to throughout the day. They often tell me that their list allows them to tackle the exercises one at a time, without feeling overwhelmed. The following list is *your* quick reference guide. You can start with just one or try them all in one session. Whatever works for you. You will benefit either way.

Before You Begin

These are exercises you can do in your home — with your doctor's permission, of course. As you start each exercise, focus on making slow, purposeful movements. If you feel dizzy, stop and sit down. If the feeling persists, consult your doctor.

Hang on to something solid if you need help with balance. If you're moving around, make sure the area is free of obstacles. Ask for help if you need it. If someone is watching you move, they can also help correct your position for optimal results. And don't forget that you're getting stronger each time you practice these exercises. Give yourself a pat on the back for taking ownership of your body.

Before we get started, can we talk about feet for a moment? I'm a barefoot soul. I much prefer to have my feet unencumbered by shoes and socks, but I know not everyone feels that way. For a variety of reasons, many of my older clients do not remove footwear to complete these exercises. As we age, the fat deposits on the soles of our feet diminish, and standing barefoot can sometimes be painful. Our circulation is reduced, which will cause feet to get —

and stay — cold quickly. While the exercises I suggest should ultimately improve circulation, you might need time to be convinced that being barefoot is beneficial. Whatever you choose, the most important thing is that you're at ease when performing the exercises. If that means leaving shoes and socks on your feet, so be it.

Definitions

As a reminder, here are some terms we discussed earlier in the book. You'll see these terms in the following exercises.

- Base of support: This refers to the area beneath you — whether you are standing or sitting — that makes contact with the surface that supports you. Reducing your base of support challenges your body's stability, as does changing your centre of gravity.
- Centre of gravity: This refers to the point in your body around which your weight is evenly distributed. When you bend your knees, your centre of gravity is lowered.
- Visual system: This is about your eyes, which provide visual input to your brain as you move through life.

- Vestibular system: This is the medical terminology for your inner ear, which processes sensory information about motion, equilibrium, and spatial orientation.
- Proprioception or somatosensory system: This is your brain's ability to sense your body's position in space.

NOTE: The Finger Follow exercise targets the visual and vestibular systems, while all of the exercises listed work the somatosensory system.

Now let's move on to the exercises.

Finger Follow

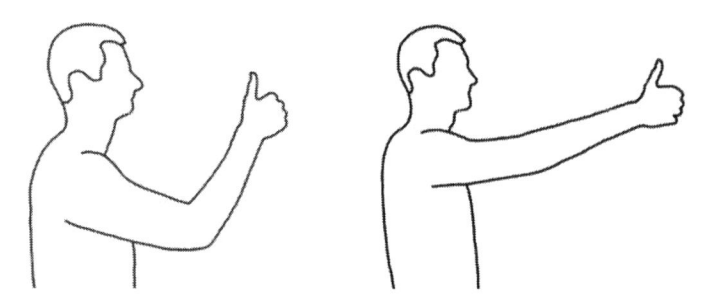

The Finger Follow is an eye-tracking exercise that helps improve balance by focusing on your visual and vestibular systems. Eye tracking exercises counteract deterioration that is a natural part of aging. The head movements will improve your ability to look around while your body is in motion throughout your day.

To start: Stand near a wall, counter, or sturdy chair and make sure you can reach it with your hand. I recommend you do this standing up, but you can also do it sitting in a chair.

Remember: If you feel dizzy during the exercise, stop, sit down, and look straight ahead until the feeling passes.

1. Visual only: Using either hand, make a fist and stick your thumb towards the sky. Lift your hand in front of your face at eye level, approximately 12 inches away. Keep your arm bent at the elbow and hold your hand in this position.

2. Side to side: Slowly move your arm to the left, watching your thumb with both eyes, without moving your head or neck. This is a small movement because only your eyes are moving. Slowly move your arm back to the middle, and then to the right, and back to the middle again — always following with just your eyes.

3. Down and up: Continue tracking your thumb with both eyes as you slowly move your arm towards the floor, then back to the middle, up to the ceiling, and back to the middle again.

4. Visual and vestibular: Do Steps 1 to 3 a second time, but this time, stretch your arm straight out in front of you with no bend at the elbow. Follow your thumb with your eyes and your head as you move your arm through the same positions: left, middle, right, middle, down, middle, up, middle.

Do you need to make it easier? Sit down to complete the finger follow.

Are you ready to make it harder? Reduce your base of support by staggering one foot in front of the other.

Static Balance

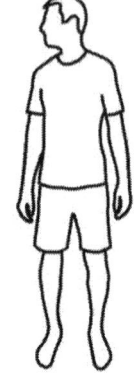

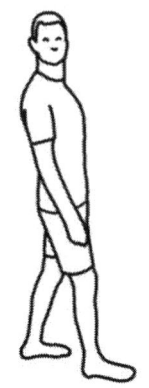

Static balance exercises work on your postural stability by decreasing your base of support and incorporating different head positions that change the orientation of your head in space. As you reduce your base of support, you want to be able to remain standing. There are five foot positions that have you moving from a wide, stable base of support to a narrower, less stable one. They are:
- Feet wide
- Feet close together
- Feet staggered forward and back at hip's width
- Feet staggered closer together with the big toe of the back foot touching the heel of the front foot
- Standing on one leg with the other foot lifted off the ground.

When you're ready to shift to a narrower base of support, I want you to remember a few things. As you reduce your base of support, take a moment to readjust your centre of gravity — you may naturally place more weight on one foot, which will unbalance you before you begin the exercise. This is normal when you're first starting out. Slowly shift your weight (your centre of gravity) so it's evenly distributed between both feet.

To start: Ideally, you'll want to try this balance challenge in bare feet. Stand beside a wall, counter, or sturdy chair and make sure you can reach it with your hand.

1. Feet wide: Begin with your feet at hip's width apart.
2. Head turn: Turn your head to one side and hold this position for 15 seconds. Remember, the position should feel challenging without making you feel like falling over. If you feel like you might fall, turn your head back to the front and stand comfortably. Take a break and sit down whenever you need a rest.
3. Position hold: If you can safely hold that position for 15 seconds, work up to holding the position for 30 seconds.
4. Narrow your base: Do the exercise again, but with your feet closer together. Begin by turning your head and holding it for 15 seconds, working up to 30 seconds.
5. Keep narrowing your base: Once you're comfortable doing the exercise in that position, it's time to reduce your base of support again. This time, stagger your feet so one foot is further ahead than the other. When you advance to the staggered heel-toe and one-foot-up positions, switch the position of your feet and try again. For example, if you started with your right foot forward and your left foot back, reverse them. If you find any of these positions too challenging, you can bend your knees to lower your centre of gravity.
6. Position hold: Continue trying to keep your head turned and hold this position for 15 to 30 seconds.
7. Head position: Try turning your head to the other side, or dropping your ear towards your shoulder instead.

Do you need to make it easier? Move through the different foot positions to reduce your base of support without moving your head. You can also stretch your arms out to the side — what I call airplane arms — to increase your base of support.

Are you ready to make it harder? Repeat the exercise with your eyes closed.

Clock Toe Taps

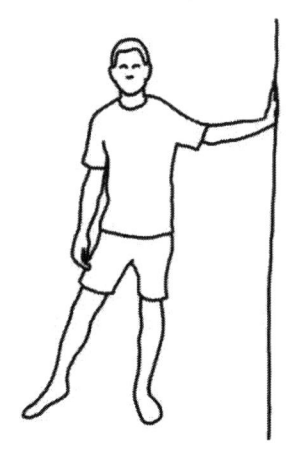

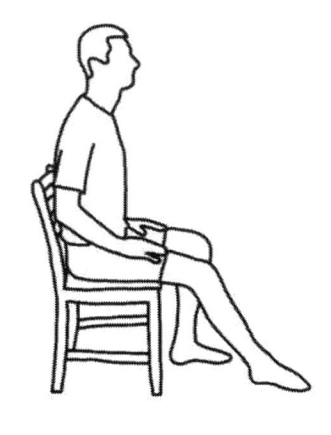

Clock toe taps are a transition exercise to help you incorporate static balance with a degree of coordination as you move one leg away from your body and back again. This exercise is more dynamic than the last balance challenge, but not as involved as a fully dynamic balance exercise.

To start: Stand near a counter, wall, or sturdy chair, and hang on with your left hand. You will be working the right leg first, so make sure there are no obstacles in a circle near your right leg. Imagine that there's a clock face on the floor and you're standing in the middle of it. The goal is to tap each hour on the clock from 12 o'clock all the way to six o'clock, and then repeat the toe taps in the opposite direction back to 12 o'clock. Try to do this exercise three times on each leg. Here's how it works:

1. Twelve o'clock: Reach your right foot forward with a straight leg and gently tap your big toe at the 12 o'clock

position, then return it to the ground beside your left foot. Keep your weight on your standing leg, and gently but quickly tap your toe on the ground.

2. Moving around the clock: Continue tapping your toe around the imaginary clock, always returning to the centre between each "hour" and placing your foot on the ground before continuing to the next "hour." If a particular position feels too difficult or uncomfortable, don't reach as far. Instead of tapping the toe on the ground, just lift the leg in that direction and return it to the centre, beside your left foot.

3. Switch legs: Once you have finished the exercise with your right leg, turn around and hold on to your support with your right hand.

4. Repeat: Repeat the toe taps with your left foot, beginning at 12 o'clock and working backwards from 11 o'clock down to six o'clock. Repeat in the opposite direction, returning to 12 o'clock.

Do you need to make it easier? Sit on the edge of a sturdy chair and perform the toe taps from 12 o'clock to three o'clock on the right leg, and from 12 o'clock to nine o'clock on the left leg. Start by doing the exercises once on each leg, and gradually work your way up to three repetitions.

Are you ready to make it harder? If you feel strong and stable enough, try a few clock toe taps without holding on to your support.

Dynamic Walking

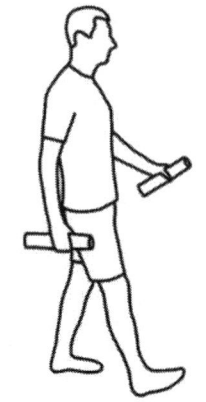

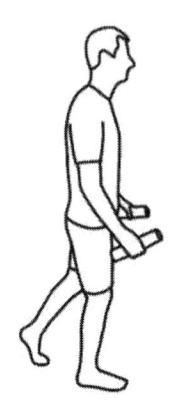

Walking is the ultimate dynamic balance challenge because you constantly shift your centre of gravity and base of support. Before you begin this exercise, make sure the surrounding area is clear of obstacles. Hallways are a great place to practice walking because the walls are close to you in case you need to steady yourself, and hallways are typically already clear spaces for moving about. If you are comfortable practicing outside, you can walk further. If you're staying indoors, make space to walk ten to 12 steps at minimum.

Equipment needed: Two empty paper towel tubes. Holding the tubes will keep your shoulders down and back, instead of rounded forward. This is a better posture for walking.

1. Tubes: Hold a tube in each hand, with your hands at hip height. One open end of the tube should face forward while the other open end faces backward. The tubes will help you keep your shoulders rotated correctly. If you feel the open end of the tube touching your leg, you've rounded your shoulders and the tubes are no longer pointing forward and back.

2. Shoulders: Drop your shoulders away from your ears as you maintain an upright posture. Imagine you're trying to slip your shoulder blades into your back pockets.

These two steps will ensure that you're aligning your bones before you begin walking.

3. Walk: To begin walking, lift one foot and bring it forward. As you lower it to the ground, use the entire foot. Plant your heel first, roll forward on to your foot, then push off the ball of your foot and big toe as you lift the other foot. This rolling movement helps propel you forward, using your leg muscles. What many people do, however, is swing their leg instead of pushing off the big toe. This movement weakens the muscles, which makes it difficult to lift that big toe up enough to clear the ground. Involving your entire body in the practice of walking properly will improve your balance and posture.

4. Arms: Engage your arms as a counterbalance. That means that when your left foot is forward, your right arm should move forward. When your right foot is forward, your left arm should move forward.

Do you need to make it easier? Skip the first two steps and go straight to Step 3, holding on to the wall with one hand as you practice planting your heel, rolling through your foot, then pushing off the front of your foot. You can also try using walking poles or some other stability device to increase your base of support and help hold you upright.

Are you ready to make it harder? Replace the paper towel tubes with light hand weights, and try to increase your walking speed.

Lower Body Strength Exercises

The following exercises are designed to strengthen your lower body. Strong muscles and bones allow us to lift our legs and feet over obstacles. All of these strengthening exercises are more effective if they're done standing up. But where possible, seated variations are included. If you choose to do these exercises standing, sit down and take a break if you need to rest.

High March

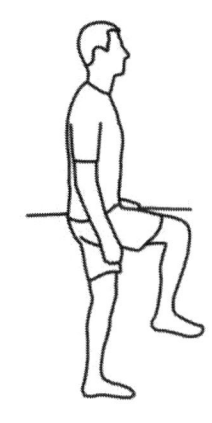

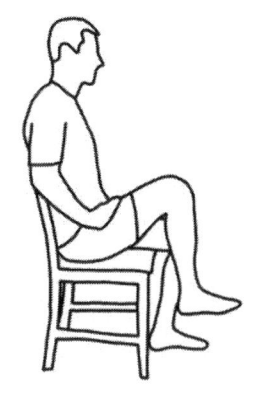

To start: Stand near a wall, counter, or sturdy chair and make sure you can reach it with your hand. Think of a soldier marching in place.

1. Lift: Lift one knee up to hip level and hold it up for three to five seconds.
2. Lower: Use control to lower the leg to the starting position. (Don't use gravity!)
3. Repeat: Repeat Steps 1 and 2 on the other leg.

Aim for ten marches, alternating sides with each repetition.

Do you need to make it easier? Sit on the edge of a sturdy chair and perform the marches in a seated position. Start with as many as you can, and work your way up to ten.

Are you ready to make it harder? Do a second set of ten marches.

Heel Raises

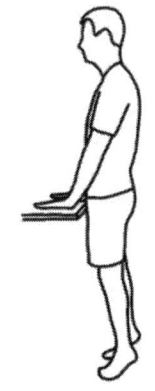

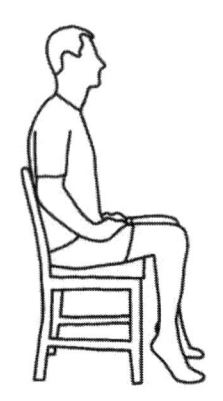

To start: Stand facing a counter, wall, or sturdy chair, hanging on with both hands.
1. Foot position: Stand tall with your feet hip's width apart.
2. Lift: Rise up onto the balls of your feet, avoiding leaning forward. Hold for 3 to 5 seconds.
3. Lower: Use control to lower to the starting position. (Don't use gravity!)

Aim for ten heel raises.

Do you need to make it easier? Sit on the edge of a sturdy chair and perform the heel raises in a seated position.

Are you ready to make it harder? Lift one foot off the ground to do one-legged heel raises. Lower your foot to the ground. Switch to the other leg and repeat.

Counter Squats

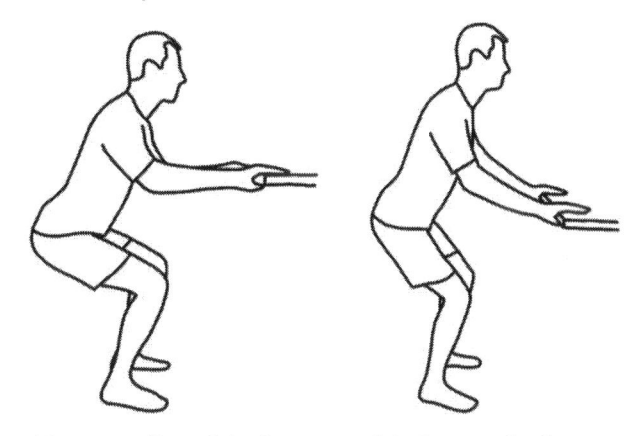

To start: Stand facing your kitchen or bathroom counter and hang on with both hands.

1. Foot position: Open your legs to shoulder-width. Try to keep your feet facing forward — including your toes and heels. If you find this position uncomfortable on your ankles, turn your toes out slightly — to 11 and one, or ten and two on a clock face.
2. Sit: Lower your bum down and back as if you're sitting in a chair. Keep your back straight, knees above your feet, and weight on your heels. Note: Your body can lean forward as you squat down, but keep your back straight as you do. Don't nosedive forward with a rounded back.
3. Stand: Push into your heels to come back up to standing.

Aim for ten counter squats.

Do you want to make it easier? Only lower hallway down, then back up (also known as a half squat).

Are you ready to make it harder? Perform it as a sit-to-stand above a chair — not hanging on to the counter. Make sure the chair is pushed against a wall so it won't move on you.

Four-Way Hip Strengthener

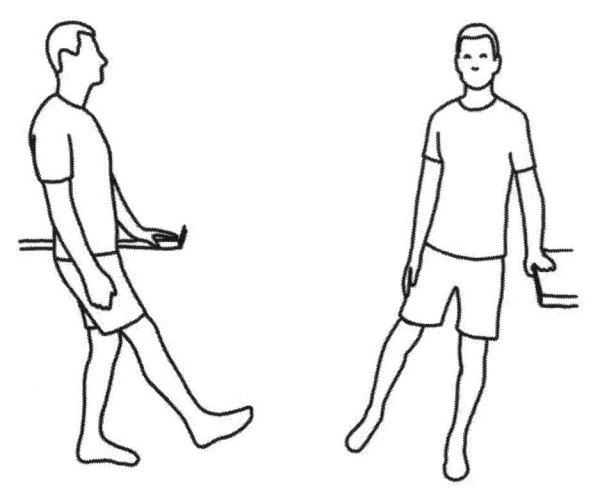

To start: Stand near a wall, counter, or sturdy chair and hang on with your right hand. You will move your left leg in four directions, so make sure you won't hit anything as you lift and lower your leg.

1. Forward: Keeping your left leg straight, slowly lift it forward and lower it just as slowly to the starting position. Don't swing it back and forth; use control to move it.
2. Side: Lift your straight leg out to the side and back to the starting position. Don't lean over to try and lift it higher.
3. Back: Squeeze your bum and lift your leg behind you and back to the starting position. Don't lean forward in an attempt to lift the leg higher.

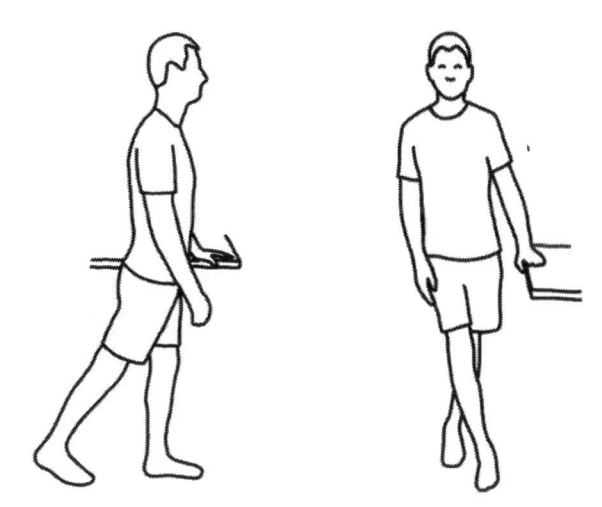

4. Across: Lift your straight leg across your standing leg and back to the starting position.

5. Repeat: Repeat the entire sequence three to five times on the same leg.

6. Other leg: To repeat on the right leg, move to the other side of the chair and hang on to the chair with your left hand. If you're hanging on to a counter or wall, turn around and hold on with your left hand. Repeat Steps 1 to 5 on your right leg.

Do you want to make it easier? Bend your knees, both on the standing leg and the working leg. Take frequent breaks and sit down to rest.

Are you ready to make it harder? Do ten repetitions in each direction before you move on to the next position.

Sideways Walking

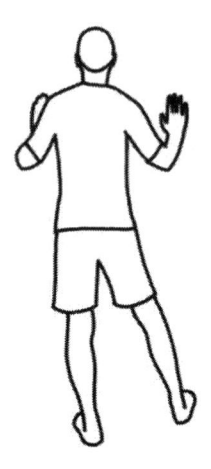

Sideways walking strengthens smaller muscles along the inside and outside of our legs and improves lower-body coordination. Before you do this exercise, check that the space to your right and left is clear of obstacles.

To start: Begin by standing up. Face the wall and place your hands on it as you begin to walk sideways.

1. Foot position: Keep your toes and heels pointed towards the wall. Look down at your feet and make sure both are pointing forwards — sometimes toes like to turn outwards.

2. Left foot: Lift your left foot and move it to the left, then place it back on the ground.

3. Right foot: Lift your right foot and move it closer to your left foot, then place it back on the

ground. Continue stepping to the left for five to ten steps. The amount of space you have will dictate how many steps you can take.

4. Change direction: Stay facing the wall to move in the other direction. Lift your right foot and move it to the right, then place it back on the ground.

5. Left foot: Lift your left foot and move it closer to your right foot, then place it back on the ground. Continue stepping to the right for five to ten steps.

Do you need to make it easier? Sit down and take a break before you change direction. Just remember to start at the same place you paused and move the other way.

Are you ready to make it harder? Keep switching directions and aim for five minutes of sideways walking.

Active Sitting

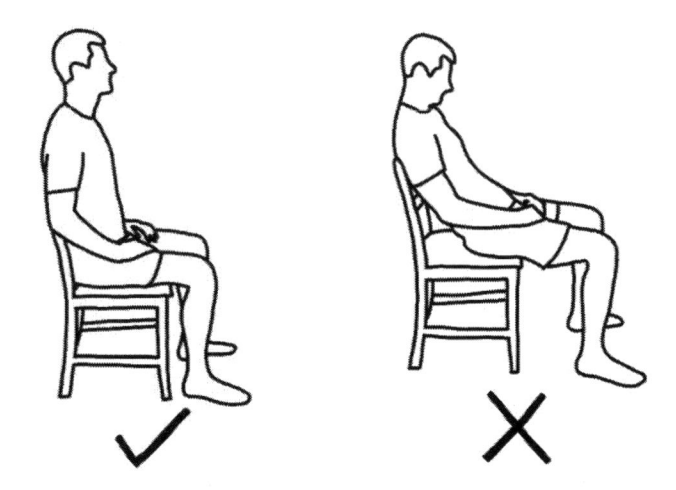

Active sitting helps us load our muscles and bones to fight the effects of gravity. Instead of outsourcing the role of our muscles by slumping in our seats, we should sit tall.

To start: Begin by sitting in a kitchen or dining room chair that has a firm seat.

1. Shifting forward: Slide your bottom forward so you're not leaning back in the chair. Place both feet flat on the floor in front of you. If your legs are shorter and you can't touch the floor, you can place a large book or block on the floor to support your feet. Don't roll onto your tailbone. Imagine you have a tail and you want the tail behind you so you can wag it. Often, people roll backwards so they're resting on their

tailbone instead of their sit bones — these are the bony part of your bum, the lower edge of your pelvis.

2. Shoulder position: Drop your shoulders away from your ears. It should feel like you're letting them slide down your back.

3. Head position: Pull your head and neck back so your ears are sitting over your shoulders, not pushed forward. Your head is now positioned over your centre of gravity, which is allowing you to strengthen your bones by loading them. Feel your muscles and bones at work.

Aim for five minutes of active sitting every hour.

Do you need to make it easier? Start with two minutes of active sitting.

Are you ready to make it harder? Try for 10 minutes of active sitting every hour.

Active Standing

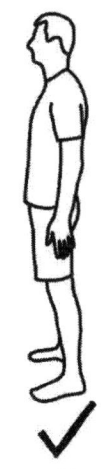

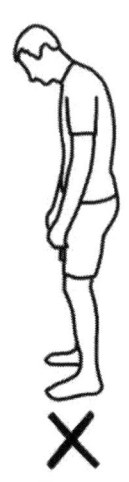

Active standing allows us to align our bones while strengthening our muscles and bones in the process. Active standing should feel like work. Your muscles are working together to hold you upright. This is a more effective way to stand, instead of dropping into your heels and hips. Resist the pull of gravity!

For this exercise, you can remove your shoes if you're willing to be bare foot.

To start: Stand up.

1. Foot position: Imagine a triangle under each foot. Instead of sinking backwards onto your heels and dropping into your hips, engage your entire foot by transferring more weight forward and across the width of your foot. Your toes and heels on both feet should be pointing forwards, not turned in or out.

2. Arm position: Allow your arms to hang smoothly at the sides of your body, not behind or in front of your torso. Your palms should be touching your thighs, not facing backwards.

3. Shoulder position: Drop your shoulders away from your ears. It should feel like you're letting them slide down your back.

4. Head position: Pull your head and neck back so your ears are sitting over your shoulders, not pushed forward. Your head is now positioned over your centre of gravity, which is allowing you to strengthen your bones by loading them. Feel your muscles and bones at work. Aim for five minutes of active standing every hour.

Do you need to make it easier? Start with two minutes of active standing.

Are you ready to make it harder? Try for 10 minutes of active standing every hour.

Joint Mobility

CARs — Controlled Articular Rotations — involve making s-l-o-w, controlled circles that increase mobility in your joints. Drawing these circles helps you feel less stiff and move more fluidly. Remember, motion is lotion!

To start: You can stand or sit for most of these exercises, unless specific instructions are provided below. If you stand, turn sideways and hang on to a sturdy support such as a wall, counter, table or chair. The key is to make slow and controlled movements. Many times, I see people drawing fast and sloppy circles. Fight the urge to get through the exercises as quickly as possible. Try to make the circular movements last for at least the number of seconds listed in the instructions.

Do you need to make it easier? Count fewer seconds to complete the joint rotations, or repeat the sequence fewer times. Take breaks and sit down for a rest. For the smaller joints in your ankles, hands, and fingers, you can move them in slow circles while you're lying in bed. You can also try to move your joints when you're sitting in a chair (except for your hips — you'll need to stand up and balance on one leg to do a full circle from the hip joint).

Please don't try to make it harder. CARs are a feel-good movement designed to keep your joints mobile. We don't want to force them to work harder, just better!

Ankles

1. Joint position: Lift your right foot off the ground and bend your knee.
2. Clockwise: Count to ten as you draw circles with your foot by rotating your ankle in a clockwise direction.
3. Counterclockwise: Count to ten as you draw circles in the opposite direction.
4. Repeat: Repeat this sequence five to ten times, then lower your right foot to the ground.
5. Other ankle: Lift your left foot off the ground and repeat the entire sequence in both directions, then lower your left foot to the ground.

You can even try wiggling your toes a little before we move on to the next joint. These aren't rotations, just an additional feel-good movement.

Knees

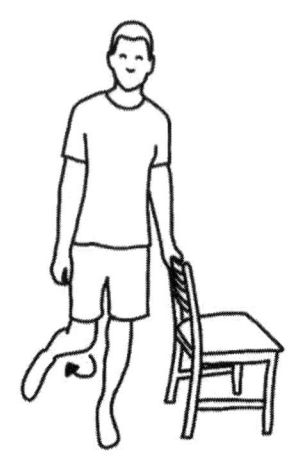

1. Joint position: Lift your right foot off the ground and bend the knee.
2. Clockwise: Count to ten as you draw circles using the lower part of your right leg — below the knee — in a clockwise direction.
3. Counterclockwise: Count to ten as you draw circles in the opposite direction.
4. Repeat: Repeat this sequence five to ten times, then lower your right foot to the ground.
5. Other knee: Lift your left foot off the ground and repeat the entire sequence. Lower your left foot to the ground.

Hips

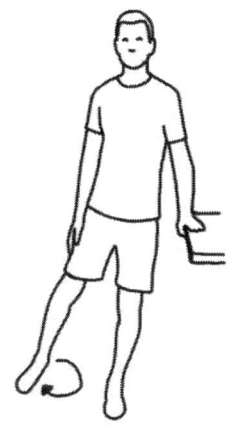

To start: The hip circles need to be completed from a standing position. Stand beside a counter, wall, or sturdy chair.

1. Joint position: Lift your right foot off the ground while holding on to your support with your left hand. You can lean on your support to do these — that way, your moving foot won't hit the ground.
2. Clockwise: Count to ten as you slowly draw circles with your leg. The movement should come from your hip socket so that you are rotating your whole leg, with your leg straight. If you find it too difficult to make circles with your leg straight, try bending your knee.
3. Counterclockwise: Count to ten again as you draw circles with your leg in the opposite direction.
4. Repeat: Repeat this sequence five to ten times, then lower your right foot to the ground.
5. Other hip: Change your body position so that you can hang on to your support with your right hand. Lift your left foot off the ground and repeat the entire sequence. Lower your left foot to the ground.

Waist

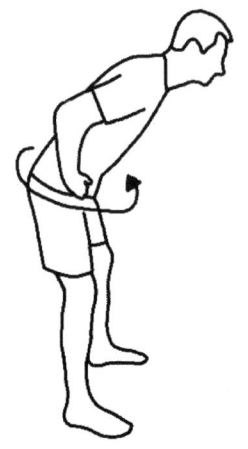

To start: If you're standing, keep your feet at hip's width. You can put your hands on your hips or stretch them out to the sides before you begin. If you want to do the waist circles sitting down, sit on the front part of the chair with your feet planted on the ground. This will give you clearance to circle towards the back without hitting the back of your chair.

1. Clockwise: Slowly rotate your upper body in a clockwise circle as you count to five.
2. Counterclockwise: Repeat in a counterclockwise circle for five more seconds.
3. Repeat: Repeat this sequence five to ten times.

The remaining exercises can be done standing or sitting.

Fingers

1. Joint position: Lift your hands in front of you and spread out your fingers. You will work both hands at the same time.
2. Clockwise: Starting with your pinky fingers, slowly draw circles with each pinky finger in a clockwise direction for five seconds.
3. Counterclockwise: Repeat in the opposite direction for five more seconds.
4. Repeat: Repeat circles in both directions with each finger. So after you have finished with your pinky fingers, move on to your ring fingers, then your middle fingers, and your index fingers. When it's time to work your thumbs, slow down the circles even more. They have a bigger range of motion, so try to make circles with them for seven to eight seconds in each direction.

Wrists

1. Joint position: Lift your hands in front of you at chest height.
2. Clockwise: Slowly rotate both of your wrists in a clockwise direction while you count to ten.
3. Counterclockwise: Slowly rotate your wrists in the opposite direction while you count to ten again.
4. Repeat: Repeat this sequence five to ten times. Lower your hands to your sides when you are finished.

Elbows

1. Joint position: Lift your arms out to the side at a slight angle. Bend your elbows so that your hands are pointing towards the floor. Your arms should look like a scarecrow.
2. Clockwise: Slowly make circles by rotating your lower arm — below the elbow — clockwise for five seconds.
3. Counterclockwise: Repeat in the other direction for another five seconds.
4. Repeat: Repeat this sequence five to ten times. Lower your arms to your sides when you are finished.

Shoulders

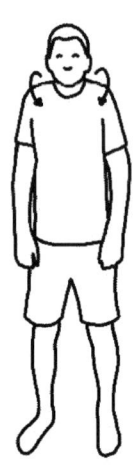

1. Joint position: Relax your shoulders and keep your arms dropped at your side.
2. Forward: Slowly roll your shoulders forward, up, back, and down as you count to five.
3. Backward: Repeat in the opposite direction: pull them down, back, up, and forward as you count another five seconds.
4. Repeat: Repeat this sequence five to ten times.

Neck

1. Clockwise: Looking straight ahead, rotate your head in a clockwise direction for five seconds. The movement should look as if you're drawing a circle with the tip of your nose.

2. Counterclockwise: Switch directions and repeat as you count another five seconds.

NOTES

1. At the beginning of life, babies crawl on all fours; children and adults walk on two feet; and older adults walk with a cane — the third leg — towards the end of life.

2. Public Health Agency of Canada, You CAN Prevent Falls! (Ottawa: Government of Canada, 2005, Revised 2015), https://www.canada.ca/en/public-health/services/health-promotion/aging-seniors/publications/publications-general-public/you-prevent-falls.html. Reprinted with permission from the Minister of Health, 2019.

3. National Council on Aging (website), Falls Prevention Facts, accessed March 22, 2019, https://www.ncoa.org/news/resources-for-reporters/get-the-facts/falls-prevention-facts/.

4. Robert Wood, "Why Seniors Fall," *Electronic Caregiver* (March 29, 2012), https://www.youtube.com/watch?v=T5x6kTrwgYw.

5 Canadian Society for Exercise Physiology (website), *Canadian Physical Activity Guidelines for Adults - 18-64 years*, accessed January 4, 2019, https://csepguidelines.ca/wp-content/uploads/2018/03/CSEP_PAGuidelines_adults_en.pdf.

6 Canadian Society for Exercise Physiology (website), *Canadian Physical Activity Guidelines for Older Adults - 65 years and older*, accessed January 4, 2019, https://csepguidelines.ca/wp-content/uploads/2018/03/CSEP_PAGuidelines_older-adults_en.pdf.

7 U.S. Department of Health and Human Services, *Physical Activity Guidelines for Americans, 2nd edition*. (Washington, DC: U.S. Department of Health and Human Services; 2018), https://health.gov/paguidelines/second-edition/pdf/Physical_Activity_Guidelines_2nd_edition.pdf.

8 Rachel C. Colley et al., "Physical activity of Canadian adults: Accelerometer results from the 2007 t0 2009 Canadian Health Measures Survey," *Health Reports* 22, no. 1 (January 2011)): 1-2, http://www.statcan.gc.ca/pub/82-003-x

/2011001/article/11396-eng.pdf.

9 Wood, "Why Seniors Fall," *Electronic Caregiver* (March 29, 2012), https://www.youtube.com/watch?v=T5x6kTrwgYw. Reprinted with permission.

10 Amanda Sterczyk, *Move More, Your Life Depends On It: Practical Tips to Add More Movement to Your Day* (Ottawa: Createspace Independent Publishing Platform, 2018).

11 Colley, "Physical activity of Canadian adults", 4. Numbers have been rounded to the nearest 100 for ease of reporting.

12 Wojtek J. Chodzko-Zajko et al., "Exercise and physical activity for older adults: Position stand," *Medicine & Science in Sports & Exercise* (July 2009): 1510-1530, DOI: 10.1249/MSS.0b013e3181a0c95c.

13 "Rating of Perceived Exertion Scale," Productive Fitness, accessed October 10, 2016, http://www.productivefitness.com/ratingofPerceivedexertion.aspx.

14 Rachel C. Colley, Isabelle Michaud and Didier Garriguet, "Reallocating time between sleep, sedentary and active behaviours: Associations with obesity and health in Canadian adults," *Health Reports* 29, no. 4 (April 18, 2018), http://www.statcan.gc.ca/pub/82-003-x/2018004/article/54951-eng.htm

15 Anthony Komaroff, "Why does balance decline with age?" Ask Dr. K/Harvard Health Publications (website), accessed September 22, 2018, https://www.askdoctork.com/why-does-balance-decline-with-age-201306054928.

16 Andrew Iwanicki, "How I felt after 70 days of lying in bed for science," *Vice Magazine*, Feb. 5, 2015, https://www.vice.com/en_us/article/jma83d/nasa-patient-8179-200.

17 Kimberly Turtenwald, "The effects of immobility on the body systems," AZCentral (website) accessed Feb 7, 2015, https://healthyliving.azcentral.com/the-effects-of-immobility-on-the-body-systems-12497238.html.

[18] Kay Lazar, "Fitness for elders is key, study finds," *Boston Globe,* January 24, 2015, https://www.bostonglobe.com/metro/2015/01/24/researchers-redouble-efforts-understand-and-improve-elders-mobility-problems/HoU5skivE2wvsGvT1H38ZO/story.html

[19] Andrew Iwanicki, "How I felt after 70 days of lying in bed for science." Reprinted with permission.

[20] The Ottawa Hospital, *How to reduce your fall risk at home* (Ottawa: The Ottawa Hospital, 2015), 1-12.

[21] Darren E.R. Warburton et al. on behalf of the PAR-Q+ Collaboration, "The Physical Activity Readiness Questionnaire for Everyone (PAR-Q+) and Electronic Physical Activity Readiness Medical Examination (ePARmedX+)," *Health & Fitness Journal of Canada,* 4, no. 2 (2011): 3-23.

[22] Physiopedia (website), Balance, accessed March 27, 2019, https://www.physio-pedia.com/Balance.

[23] Barry Franklin and Robert Sweetgall, *One Heart, Two Feet: Enhancing Heart Health, One Step at a Time* (Clayton, MO: Creative Walking, 2016), 60. Reprinted with permission.

[24] World Health Organization, *Fact Sheet on Physical Activity*, https://www.who.int/news-room/fact-sheets/detail/physical-activity. Reprinted with permission.

[25] Meg Selig, "Is it true that 'Movement is medicine'?," *Psychology Today*, March 30, 2017, https://www.psychologytoday.com/us/blog/changepower/201703/is-it-true-movement-is-medicine.

[26] Excerpt from an interview with Cassandra McCoy, ATC, LAT, conducted via video chat and email on April 6, 2019.

[27] Amanda Sterczyk, *Move More, Your Life Depends On It: Practical Tips to Add More Movement to Your Day* (Ottawa: CreateSpace Independent Publishing Platform, 2018).

ACKNOWLEDGEMENTS

To Mary Yoke, thank you for your inspiring words in your ACSM 2017 conference presentation. You vocalized what I had been thinking for years — that the fitness industry is not serving a large segment of our population. These are the individuals who will never step foot in a gym or group fitness class, do not meet the minimum recommendations for physical activity, but still want someone to help them achieve their personal fitness goals.

To Cassandra McCoy, thank you for fitting our interview into your incredibly busy life. You are a superhero!

To Bob Wood, thank you for agreeing to write the foreword to this book. Your enthusiasm and support of my work is so appreciated.

To my editorial team:
    Kaarina Stiff
    Dianna Little
    Emily Sterczyk
    Matthew Bin
    Rhys Jennings

Thank you for your hard work and professionalism in helping me get my book into the world.

To my family, thank you for your support of my "Bevolution."

To my clients, thank you for entrusting me with your fitness goals. I love working with all of you.

REVIEWS OF *MOVE MORE, YOUR LIFE DEPENDS ON IT*

"*Move More* contains simple and powerful tips I have incorporated into my daily life. This book ranks as one of my favorites. The information is inspiring, timeless, well-organized, and an easy read. Amanda does a great job sharing her knowledge in a fun way."

— Fabiana Meredith, co-founder Qi

"As a teacher and musician, I suffer from several repetitive strain injuries and back problems related to performance. *Move More, Your Life Depends On It* is a huge wake up call for so many of us who live our lives behind a computer and think there isn't any opportunity in our daily routine to exercise. Amanda's book showed me that there are countless opportunities throughout each day to exercise and reduce some of the chronic pain I experience just by doing my daily tasks. I highly recommend it for anyone in any industry."

— Danielle Allard, singer/songwriter

"Amanda's language is both humorous and serious. It feels like a friend is talking to you about something she is really excited to share. The tone made this book fun to read, and it was never dull or dry...I have an increased awareness of and motivation for fitting in little snacks of movement throughout my day."

— Lauren

"Absolutely loved Amanda's style of writing and her excellent and simple idea to help anyone become more active! I will definitely be recommending this book!"

— Colin

"Excellent book, easy to read, very good for seniors or anyone who needs to add move movement in their daily life."

— Amazon customer

ABOUT THE AUTHOR

Amanda Sterczyk is an author and certified personal trainer based in Ottawa, Canada. In 2016, she founded The Move More Institute™, an initiative to promote healthy active living and teach individuals how to sneak exercise into their daily lives. Her slogan is "Move more, feel better." Amanda holds a Master's degree in social psychology from Carleton University. Her first book, *Move More, Your Life Depends On It: Practical Tips to Add More Movement to Your Day* was published in 2018.

You can connect with Amanda online by visiting her website:

http://www.amandasterczyk.com

Made in the USA
Middletown, DE
19 May 2020